AND WE FLY AWAY

LIVING BEYOND ALZHEIMER'S

RAY ASHFORD

Augsburg Books
MINNEAPOLIS

AND WE FLY AWAY
Living beyond Alzheimer's

Copyright © 2003 Ray Ashford. All rights reserved. Except for brief quotations in critical articles or reviews, no part of this book may be reproduced in any manner without prior written permission from the publisher. Write to: Permissions, Augsburg Fortress, Box 1209, Minneapolis, MN 55440.

Large-quantity purchases or custom editions of this book are available at a discount from the publisher. For more information, contact the sales department at Augsburg Fortress, Publishers, 1-800-328-4648, or write to: Sales Director, Augsburg Fortress, Publishers, P.O. Box 1209, Minneapolis, MN 55440-1209.

Bible quotations marked KJV are from the King James Version of the Bible.

Bible quotations marked RSV are from the Revised Standard Version of the Bible, copyright © 1946, 1952, 1971 by the Division of Christian Education of the National Council of the Churches of Christ in the USA. Used by permission.

Bible quotations marked NRSV are from the New Revised Standard Version of the Bible, copyright © 1989 by the Division of Christian Education of the National Council of the Churches of Christ in the USA. Used by permission.

Excerpt from *The Prophet* by Kahlil Gibran, copyright © 1923 by Kahlil Gibran and renewed 1951 by Administrators C.T.A. of Kahlil Gibran Estate and Mary G. Gibran. Use by permission of Alfred A. Knopf, a division of Random House, Inc.

Excerpt from *The Weight of Glory* by C.S. Lewis copyright © C.S. Lewis Pte. Ltd. 1949. Extract reprinted by permission.

"The Heavenly City" by Stevie Smith, from *The Collected Poems of Stevie Smith* (New York: Oxford University Press, 1976), p. 43.

"Autumn" by Rainer Maria Rilke, from *Fifty Selected Poems,* C.F. MacIntyre, trans. (Berkeley and San Francisco: University of California Press, 1941), p.43.

Excerpt from Robert Farrar Capon, *The Parables of Grace* (Grand Rapids: William B. Eerdman's Publishing Co., 1988), p. 106, now published as part of Kingdom, Grace, Judgment.

Library of Congress Cataloging-in-Publication Data
Ashford, Ray.
  And we fly away: living beyond Alzheimer's / Ray Ashford.
   p. cm.
Includes bibliographical references
ISBN 0-8066-4570-9 (pbk.)
  1. Consolation. 2. Ashford, Ray. 3. Bereavement—Religious aspects—Christianity. 4. Ashford, Phyllis Sharpe—Death and burial. 5. Alzheimer's disease—Religious aspects—Christianity. I. Title.
BV4905.3A84 2003
248.8'66'092—dc21   2003004509

Cover design by Marti Naughton; cover art from Getty Images; book design by Michelle L. N. Cook

The paper used in this publication meets the minimum requirements of American National Standard for Information Sciences— Permanence of Paper for Printed Library Materials, ANSI Z329.48-1984. ♾ ™

Manufactured in the U.S.A.

| 07 | 06 | 05 | 04 | 03 | 1 | 2 | 3 | 4 | 5 | 6 | 7 | 8 | 9 | 10 |

The years of our life are threescore and ten,
or even by reason of strength fourscore . . .
they are soon gone, and we fly away . . .
So teach us to number our days
that we may get a heart of wisdom.

—Psalm 90:10, 12 RSV

Contents

Prologue: Genesis   7

Part One: Elegy   11

Part Two: Healing   33

Part Three: Dawn   59

Notes   79

PROLOGUE

Genesis

In my bedroom is a picture I cherish, a head-and-shoulders photo of a solemn little girl, aged about six, with straight blonde hair cut short and a big elaborate bow perched on top of her head. She is a beautiful child, but there is, I think, more than conventional prettiness in that young face; there is also great sweetness; there is gentleness, kindness, grace.

Decades ago, about the time that picture was taken, our paths perhaps crossed, hers and mine. My parents and their three sons, myself included, had just returned to Canada after five years in India. We were visiting in the little town of Newcastle, New Brunswick, where my grandmother lived, my father's widowed mother. She was tall and thin, ever so proper, even severe, dressed entirely in black, and, I gathered, the most devoutly religious person in town. I found her intimidating.

Someone I did not meet, another Newcastle resident, was the little girl, my own age, whose picture is now in my bedroom. Her name? Phyllis Sharpe. No, we never came face to face, but who knows? Perhaps we saw each other in the drugstore, at the post office, on the beach.

If so, I wonder how I would have felt had some all-seeing person said to me, "See that little girl over there? Someday she is going to be your wife."

It was, for me, a new university, a place where I knew no one, not a soul. Discharged from the Navy, I had spent three-and-a-half days crossing the country by train, day coach all the way, and had taken a seat in the back row of a small lecture theater. It was my first day of classes and my first class of the day.

Seated immediately in front of me, as it happened, was a slim, beautiful girl with long blonde hair. I watched her talking with others before the professor's arrival. I watched her ease, her warmth, her evident kindness, and was charmed.

I first met Phyllis, actually met her, a couple of weeks later at an informal dance on campus. I crossed the hall and asked her to dance. (Perry Como, recorded, was singing "Prisoner of Love.")

As we danced, I was amazed to learn that she had been raised in Newcastle, not far away, my father's birthplace. Clearly, we had something in common, the same geography in our background! By the time our one dance was over, I was more than charmed; I was captivated.

Came the next morning and I nosed around, only to learn, disappointingly, that she already had a boyfriend, a varsity athlete. My hopes were dashed. It seemed a lost cause. But then one day, a couple of weeks later and more than a little nervously, I took a chance: I phoned and asked for a date. Much to my surprise, she said, "Yes, I'd love to go." I was so elated I felt like going out and yodeling my joy to the moon.

Two-and-a-half years later, both aged twenty-two, we were married. It was a joyous day, the best day of my life.

PART ONE

Elegy

Our life was sweeter than ever, but there were worrisome signs, signs that had been there slightly but increasingly for some years: the failing memory, the fumbling for words, the faltering judgment.

After putting it off for almost a year, Phyllis made an appointment with our family doctor. Merril questioned and listened, then referred her to a specialist. Tests followed, eight weeks of testing. That behind, we drove through a vicious snowstorm, eleven days before Christmas, to receive the results.

It was devastating news. It was dementia, probably a combination of Alzheimer's Disease and multi-infarct dementia, an ongoing series of small strokes. (Short of an autopsy, we were told, a precise diagnosis was impossible.) We drove home dazed, almost disbelieving. *It can't be*, I thought. *It can't be!* At the same time, though, I knew the truth was unavoidable, the end now inevitable.

After the initial blow came the tears. Again and again I looked at this lovely woman who had been my wife for forty-seven years; I looked at her, realizing on the one hand the extraordinary richness of our relationship over all that time and, on the other, the gradual disintegration, possibly even the horror, for which we were heading. I looked at her through a film of tears and was unable to speak.

As for Phyllis, there was sadness, yes, but not for long. A day or two later the dominant mood was one of an amazing matter-of-factness, that and a transcendent grace.

We went to church on Sunday morning, the third Sunday in Advent and less than three days after we had heard the grim news. I was unable to sing the first hymn—I was too close to tears. By my side, though, Phyllis was caroling:

> Joy to the world! The Lord is come.
> Let earth receive her King!
> Let every heart prepare him room
> And heaven and nature sing.

I was dumbfounded. Rejoice and sing? Impossible. Still, here was my wife, dying of dementia, yet singing with all her heart, in a sense singing a single triumphant word: *Yes!*

That evening, we watched a televised program of Christmas music coming from Boston's Symphony Hall. Included in the concert was an exuberant medley of carols, Cajun style. Momentarily out in the kitchen, Phyllis heard the music and returned to the den, returned dancing, no less, dancing in a spirit of sheer joy.

A word came to my mind, a word with obvious theological implications: *irrepressible*.

$\mathcal{L}$istening to the radio on Boxing Day, I happened to hear Kathleen Ferrier—a magnificently gifted person, her own life cut tragically short—singing the achingly beautiful aria from Gluck's *Orfeo and Euridice*: "What is life to me without thee? What is left if thou art dead? . . . What is life without my love?" Again there were tears.

$\mathcal{A}$ marvel to me
is how two persons wedded
can after decades
be so fused, so welded.

$\mathcal{H}$e was a mallard, she his mate. He was alive, she dead. I saw them as I was out walking, saw them at the water's edge, only a few feet away. He was standing guard over her body, her head submerged. I sensed that he was immensely weary and sad. I stopped and wondered. How many years had they been mated? How many migrations had they made, how many miles flown together? How many ducklings had they raised? In their own way, had they rejoiced and dreamed and remembered? What lay ahead for him?

He looked at me for almost a minute, wondering perhaps if I would do him harm, then swiveled his head, buried his bill in the feathers of his back and closed his eyes.

Wishing I could somehow comfort him, I walked on, shaken and sad.

*H*er life is waning, yet, saying grace,
her voice so rings with praise
that I am in awe.

*I*t was a spectacular setting, an oceanside walkway with the snow-capped Olympics sprawled across the horizon on the far side of the Strait. Walking with my love, I noticed yet again that person after person smiled and said hello.

How to account for all the friendliness? Easy. Phyllis herself. Her radiance, her warmth. She *glows* and the world glows back.

I see a pair of doves perched companionably on an overhead wire and momentarily I mourn the loss of the soaring companionship with which we were blessed until this horror began bearing you away.

Her dementia by now well advanced, my beloved and I were walking along the lakeshore on a sun-drenched summer morning when I heard her murmur something.

"What did you say?" I asked.

There was a pause, then the quiet reply: "I said, 'God, your world is beautiful.'"

We married young,
I never dreaming
our union could
bless so deeply nor,
at death's bidding,
break my heart.

$\mathcal{A}$s we were walking, there was a calamity: Phyllis fell, fractured her pelvis, and was rushed to the hospital.

Especially in those first few days, the pain was cruel. Never once, though, did I hear even a whisper of bitterness or despair, never see anything but acceptance and grace.

On one of those days, in talking with a close friend, I was lamenting the massive misfortunes that had befallen my beloved, the now disabled body and the relentlessly diminishing mind. "I could weep," I said, "when I think of how little of her is left."

His reply was unforgettable. "I understand," he said, "but it occurs to me that when you take away most of a diamond, you still have a diamond left."

I asked, "Will you be my friend in heaven?"
She looked at me and smiled. "Yes."
"That," I said, "will make heaven perfect."
Again she smiled.

$\mathcal{Y}$es, dementia has effectively destroyed much of the person I so deeply love; much of her has gone. But gone where? Into nothingness? Into oblivion?

No, I can't believe that. I believe rather in a God who loves the whole of creation so much that that same God will not permit the loss of even the smallest particle of matter, much less a human soul.

Or, I wonder, even part of a soul? Could it be, I wonder, that the part of my beloved that has gone has merely *gone on ahead* and, there, in that eternal dimension, is awaiting the remnants I still can see, is awaiting that triumphant day when once more she will be whole, entire, complete?

$\mathcal{I}$t had been a quiet, pleasant outing. A few errands, a cup of coffee, and half an hour parked down by the lake, listening to the radio and looking out over the water.

I took her back to the Manor in the late afternoon. In her room I switched on the radio, picking up the program we had been listening to in the car, and we talked for a time.

I stood to leave, but there was the music—easy, gentle, irresistible. I held out my arms and, wordlessly, she moved into them. We danced.

I looked down at her. She was smiling, delighted. Not I. A painful thought had flashed through my mind. I wondered if, after fifty-four years of dancing, this might not be the last dance of our life. I was close to tears.

Even after four years, I continue to mourn my beloved's relentless decline. Each day still, at some point in the day, the thought of her brings tears to my eyes.

I wonder, though, if vicarious suffering can relieve suffering itself. I wonder if in my sorrow, in some unfathomable way, I am easing her woes even slightly. Could it be?

I hope so.

Long ago I was vaguely interested in becoming a monk. I thought, *Wouldn't it be nice? The quietness, the simplicity, the holiness even.*

Now, decades later, I am an old man and finally, in a sense, the person I once thought of being. With my beloved in the gentle care of nurses and nuns, her life gradually ebbing away, I am now alone, quiet, celibate, and even on the way to becoming, if only in a small way, a bit of a contemplative.

Is it better, this new life? No, definitely not. But it is, thank God, introducing me to heights and depths I have never known, and for that I am most grateful.

$\mathcal{W}$e were alone in a back pew in the Manor's dusky, soaring chapel. We sat there, holding hands and saying not a word, simply absorbing the mystery, the beauty, the peace.

After a time I said the Lord's Prayer, then a brief personal prayer for ourselves, our family, the world.

A minute or two passed and I asked quietly, "Do you like this place?"

She corrected me: "I *love* this place."

There are depths, it seems, that are still intact—and, I suspect, may well remain so as long as she lives.

$\mathcal{I}$ pray for her again and again: "Please, God, grant her your peace and carry her gently Home."

Often, too, I remind myself that she has been blessed for almost seventy years with a warm beauty, a fine mind, and a rare soul; that she is blessed in her dying, blessed with a wealth of compassionate care and, still, moments of joy; that she will be blessed one day, a shining, transcendent being in an infinity of love.

Dag Hammarskjöld said it beautifully:

> For what has been—thanks!
> For what shall be—yes![1]

$\mathcal{M}$aureen, one of the head nurses, told me that yesterday Phyllis came to her and, after some groping, managed to say, "I need you." She took Maureen by the hand, led her down the hall until they came to Effie's room and there, through the open door, pointed to Effie, slumped in her wheelchair and clearly ill. Maureen went on to praise my wife's immense kindness.

I went then to see my beloved. For the first time, she could not remember my name.

Later in the day I talked with a close friend who said, "It must be hard, seeing such a dear person die by inches." It is indeed.

$\mathcal{Y}$es, there is guilt. I regret, I deeply regret, that I was not a better husband and father. I wish I had been more kind.

I wish, too, that our lives were again more equal, more balanced. It grieves me that hers is now so diminished. It grieves me that the pleasures we once enjoyed—music, conversation, walking, friends, travel, worship—are for her no longer possible.

Please, God, let there be compensation. Whether today or tomorrow, whether here or there, let there be some sublime compensation.

As I entered her room, she rose from her chair and, wordlessly, moved toward me, her arms outstretched in welcome and her face radiant, almost incandescent, with warmth and love.

I was dazzled. Even after more than fifty years of marriage, I thought I had never seen her so beautiful.

Dear God, let that moment, that picture, be with me as long as I live.

$\mathcal{D}$ementia has gradually dimmed her once fine mind. Speech, memory, and comprehension are now almost gone, yet she remains what she has been all her life, kindness personified.

We stood waiting for an elevator to take us up to the next floor, I holding her left hand and looking impatiently at the elevator's floor indicator, wondering why the delay.

At one point, though, I shifted my gaze. I looked at my wife, saw in her face only patience and calm, and saw as well, on her right and in a wheelchair, a serious disabled older woman, also waiting for the elevator. I saw also my beloved, gently stroking the older woman's forearm as it rested on the arm of her wheelchair.

True, she could no longer offer words, for the words were no longer there, but there was something she could offer, and did: a soothing touch, a moment of pure comfort.

I am helped
in reminding myself,
Yes, Today is difficult but
behind is a long golden Yesterday
and beyond is
a sublime Tomorrow.

After our visit, she walked with me to the stairwell. We kissed good-bye, and I watched her walking away. She walks slowly now, laboriously. It was a painful sight.

As I watched, I saw her pass the rooms of bed-ridden people, friends, but friends now with whom she is unable to speak; speech has all but deserted her. I watched her, in passing their rooms, gently waving to them, almost a benediction, then plodding on, plodding down the long corridor and back to the quiet of her room.

Yet again I was touched by her towering kindness, present still in spite of the massive diminishment. I was close to tears.

It suddenly dawns on me, and powerfully so, that perhaps something of what Phyllis once was, the entire and superlative person, has not been forever lost in the dark mists of dementia; perhaps that much larger part of her is still here, is part of a larger presence, a love, that is without and within me wherever I go.

I went to see her, as I do each day, but this time she was not in her room. Where was she? After looking all over the building, I finally found her—perhaps not surprisingly—alone in the chapel.

I stood at the back for a moment and watched her, seated a few pews ahead of me and still as a statue. I thought of that poor vestigial mind and ached for her, but I thought also of that magnificent soul still blessed, it seemed, with a sense of the eternal, and my heart went out to her in a rush of love. I went forward, sat down beside her, took her hand and melted inwardly at the sight of her smile.

Later, in the cafeteria, we drank ginger ale and shared a bag of potato chips. As usual, she chose the small, broken chips for herself, leaving the larger ones for me. *Here she is*, I thought, *her mind in ruins, and yet she remains unselfishness through and through*.

I found her in one of the nursing home's lounges. Along with a few others, she was watching an old black-and-white movie on television. A tenor was singing a Christmas carol.

I walked over, stood beside her and, incredulously, heard her singing quietly along, singing beautifully:

> O come, all ye faithful, joyful and triumphant,
> O come ye, O come ye to Bethlehem . . .

I was dumbfounded. Here she was, mind and memory almost gone, yet somehow drawing on profound reserves and singing still. My eyes filled with tears.

Speech now has largely disappeared, as have comprehension and memory. Her kindness, though, is unchanging, an eternal constant.

A nurse told me yesterday that, in passing, she happened to look into Margaret's room. Margaret was in there, weeping. Phyllis was also there, her arms around Margaret and, though wordlessly, offering all the comfort she could.

Said the nurse of my wife, "She is such a kind person!"

I know. I have known it for more than fifty years.

It is a fact that the last six years have been the most punishing of my life, the most punishing by far, but it is also a fact that they have been the richest, the most fertile time in my life.

How so? I have been given insights into heights and depths that earlier I never even glimpsed. I have come to see more, feel more, believe more, care more. Yes, even in all the pain I have been immeasurably blessed.

I can account for this paradoxical phenomenon only in terms of a marvelous compensatory Grace at the very heart of all of life.

"O God, my God," said Thomas Merton, "the night has values that the day never dreamed of."[2]

While she can no longer speak at any length—she is capable now only of an occasional word or two—there is a form of speech she still can manage: she can echo the words of others, a brief sentence perhaps, a phrase here and there.

More than once I have commiserated with her: "It's a tough time, sweetheart, isn't it?"

She has agreed: "A tough time."

It is as close to complaint as I have ever heard her come. "A tough time."

I am repeatedly blessed by the timeless words of Juliana of Norwich:

> But all shall be well
> and all shall be well
> and all manner of thing shall be well.[3]

Dementia has taken a massive toll. My beloved is a mere remnant of the person she was. Once a vital, glowing person, she is now stooped, feeble, all but speechless and, it seems, largely uncomprehending.

Amazingly, though, there is never a hint of restlessness or distress. There is only acceptance, steadiness, calm.

Today, as I often do, I wheeled her to the cafeteria for a time, then out into the garden and finally into the chapel before taking her back to her room.

There I sat in a pew next to the aisle and she in her wheelchair by my side. We held hands and after several minutes of silence I said aloud a brief prayer, then the Lord's Prayer, and finally the first verse and refrain of the beloved old children's hymn, "Jesus loves me," but pluralizing the refrain:

Yes, Jesus loves us,
yes, Jesus loves us,
yes, Jesus loves us,
the Bible tells us so.

Through it all, Phyllis said not a word, but I noticed that during the lines of the refrain, "Jesus loves us," she was slowly nodding her head in assent.

I marveled. Here she was, mind and memory almost gone, yet faith apparently singing still. At the same time, though, I wondered if this was the last expression of faith I would see. Possibly so. But of this I am sure: there will be faith in the invisible depths, faith in some form, as long as she lives.

Could it be that the deeper sense of God with which I seem to have been blessed in these painful years is, in part, my beloved's last great gift to a husband she has already blessed beyond telling?

Entering the Manor, I saw Sister Joan, one of my favorites. We talked briefly. Speaking of my beloved, she said sadly, "She's slipping—you know that, don't you?"

"Yes, I see it every day."

Upstairs in Phyllis's room, I sat at her bedside, held her hand, stroked her arm, watched her sleep. But then, a half hour or so later, I was amazed to see her waken *beaming*, waken in a mood of sheer elation, a mood I hadn't seen in months or even years. Her face aglow, she held both of my hands in hers, squeezing tightly from time to time, and inched forward on the pillow, getting as close as she could.

I said, "I sense you're so happy, love, you feel you could burst. Is that right?"

Much to my surprise—for questions now were almost never answered—she whispered, "Yes, yes!"

And so it continued for the whole of our visit. What triggered her euphoria? I have no idea. Will I ever see it again? Perhaps not. But thank God, thank God for transcendent moments, thank God for memory.

1 was alone in my dream, walking downhill along a glistening new highway through mountainous country. Devoid of all traffic, it was a road still without yellow lines and guard rails, a road with its unused asphalt still jet black and shiny, even glassy in spots. I was walking carefully, slipping from time to time and mindful always that immediately to my right, only a few yards away, was a great cliff falling down to dark, ominous depths. Somehow, though, I sensed that in the distance, in some beautiful valley perhaps, was my destination, some beckoning haven.

Then suddenly Phyllis appeared silently, coming up from behind me but moving in an extraordinary way, almost as if she were skating. Amazed, I saw her gliding swiftly inward and outward, at one point swooping out dangerously close to the highway's edge, then back again, then racing, weaving downhill, farther and farther away, doubtless on her way to a place we would someday share, our journey's end.

I wakened.

Two weeks later, two weeks to the day, I went as usual to see her in the afternoon. As she slept, I sat at her bedside, held her hand, leaned over and kissed her from time to time. I also said an occasional few words, hoping, I suppose, even half believing, that there might be some response at the deepest of levels.

Among those words, I told her about my dream and said also, "Someday soon, my dearest, you'll be leaving me and moving on into the life beyond. They'll all be there to greet you—Tim, your mother and father, my parents as well, Aunt Min and Grandma Giles, they and a host of friends. Not only that, but you'll be well there, wonderfully well, and one day I'll join you."

After a time, she wakened, though not entirely. She seemed distant, unseeing. I stayed for a time, said a prayer, then rose to kiss her once again and say goodbye. Half turning her head, she watched me leave the room. Her eyes, more focused now, tracked me right to the door. It was a look I may never forget, a look implicit with . . . with what? With longing? With love? I wish I knew.

In the early evening, she was prepared for bed. There she laid her head down on the pillow, took two deep breaths, and quietly passed on.

Her death—no, her liberation—was as gentle, as graceful as the whole of her life.

> We shall rest and we shall see,
> we shall see and we shall love,
> we shall love and we shall praise,
> in the end which is no end.
> —St. Augustine[4]

PART TWO

Healing

$\mathcal{H}$er memorial service was one of great gladness. It was a time in which the lessons and prayers were a voice of vast hope, a time in which my brother Glenn paid eloquent tribute to a beloved soul, a time in which a large congregation lifted its heart to the heavens in hymns ringing with joy.

There were tears, yes—an understandable derivative of loss—but the tears were a trickle compared with the flood of praise: praise for a beautiful life, praise for a punishing but magnificent departure, and praise also for a transcendent liberation.

At the subsequent reception, the gladness continued. People sipped their tea, nibbled on sandwiches and cookies, chatted happily with friends, and stayed on, apparently reluctant to leave. Several commented that the service itself had been one they would never forget. Said a friend with tears in her eyes, "It was magnificent!"

In the evening, at an extended family gathering, the dominant mood was—still—joy. Phyllis, I know, would have been delighted. In fact, at one point in the evening I wondered if she might not have somehow had a hand in orchestrating the mood of the whole glowing day. Who knows?

On the day after her death, it dawned on me: *I believe that she is in God. I believe also that God is here. Therefore, wonder of wonders, she too is here.*

It was more, though, than a merely theological recognition, for there came also a vital awareness, a conviction at the deepest level of my being: *She is gone, truly gone, and she is free, magnificently free, and she is here, "Closer than breathing, and nearer than hands and feet." She is gone, free, here!*

Two major reconciliations occurred in our clan, one immediately before and one immediately after her passing.

Did she in some unfathomable way have a hand in both of those happy outcomes? Perhaps so. She was a peacemaker all her life and, for all I know, is a peacemaker still.

Words I have cherished for years, words that often come to mind, especially in sad and difficult times, are these, Elie Wiesel's tale of a small group of Jewish exiles left in the desert without food and drink:

One evening they collapsed with fatigue. They were four to fall asleep; they were three to rise. The father dug a grave for his wife, and the children recited the Kaddish. And they took up their walk again.

The next day they were three to lie down; only two woke up. The father dug up a grave for his older son and recited the Kaddish. And with his remaining son he continued the march.

Then one night the two stretched out. But at dawn only the father opened his eyes. He dug a grave in the sand and this is how he addressed God: "Master of the Universe, I know what You want—I understand what you are doing. You want despair to overwhelm me. You want me to cease believing in You, to cease praying to you, to cease invoking Your name to glorify and sanctify it. Well, I tell You: No, no—a thousand times No! You shall not succeed! In spite of me and in spite of You, I shall shout the Kaddish, which is a song of faith, for You and against You. This song You shall not still, God of Israel."[1]

Though he slay me, yet will I trust in him.
—Job 13:15 KJV

It is a traditional view, but no one perhaps has given it more eloquent expression than an anguished Feodor Dostoevsky, the Russian novelist, after the death of his wife, Maria.

God has designed us for infinite glory, Dostoevsky maintained, but death prevents the fulfillment of the Creator's intentions. Even the saints are struck down before they become the ultimate beings that God envisions.

Does this mean that God has been defeated? Does it mean that death is the final arbiter in determining the quality of our lives? No, for it is God, not death, who finally rules.

Accordingly, God has established that after death has had its day, there is more of life; there is life beyond death, a life wherein God has all eternity for molding us into the angelic souls we are intended to be.

Prior to her death, I wept. For six years there were tears. Altogether there was a river of tears.

Since her passing, though, there has been a difference: there has been sorrow—in fact, not a day, not even the best of days, has been without its heartache—but the actual tears have been few. Most of the pain was experienced, it seems, most of the grieving done, in those six long, punishing years.

$\mathcal{F}$or you have delivered my soul from death,
my eyes from tears,
my feet from stumbling.
I walk before the Lord
in the land of the living.
—Psalm 116:8-9 NRSV

$\mathcal{I}$ have long thought of heaven as a reality, if not a place, that is both *there*—elsewhere, distant ("transcendent," a theologian might say)—and *here*—nearby, close at hand ("immanent").

Correspondingly, I now find myself thinking of my beloved as being *there*—in some entirely different and infinitely beautiful dimension, utterly incomprehensible to my finite mind—and at the same time wonderfully *here*.

$\mathcal{1}$ remember Warren, who, all through a long and beautiful life, loved music. Shortly before he died, he wakened, beaming, and whispered to his wife, "Jessie, the music, the music! Oh, Jessie, it was sublime!"

I remember Neil, who died at the age of thirty-three, only eight months after he and Marie had been married. In the last hours of his life, Marie said, Neil's breathing became more labored and his sight began to fail. Clearly, he was slipping away. But then suddenly he sat up, something he had not done in days. His face aglow, he seemed to be gazing into infinity. "I'm going, I'm going," he said, his voice perfectly clear. There was a pause, then, "It's so beautiful over there. Beautiful!" He sank back onto the pillow and died.

"At that moment," said Marie, "something came out of him and around me, just like a pair of arms. It was so comforting, so reassuring. It was like being cradled in love. I'll never forget it."

$\mathcal{T}$he three most helpful exercises in my bereavement are walking, kindness, and prayer.

To repeat: walking, kindness, prayer. These three are lifesavers, literally; they preserve my life, my health, my sanity, and whatever I have of grace.

1 dreamed of her last night, on toward morning. I dreamed that I was cleaning up the apartment and, in the process, washing a small mountain of bedding and clothes—load after load was being put through the washer and dryer—and she was with me, close at hand. I never actually *saw* her—perhaps I was too intent on what I was doing—but she was unmistakably present and, typically, helping out, backing me up.

There was little conversation. In fact, in all the busyness I remember her saying only one thing: "I have my mind again."

"I know, sweetheart," I said. "I know."

Before long I wakened, wakened to the sound of freezing rain pattering on the window. I stumbled to the bathroom and back to bed, but, deeply moved by my dream, slept no more.

1n Celtic mythology there are references to "thin places"—a certain meadow perhaps, a hilltop, a shrine—places where there is little between the finite and the infinite, places where one is most likely to experience a heightened sense of the eternal.

"To seek such places," said Peter Gomes, "is the vocation of the wise and the good, and those who find them find the clearest communication between the temporal and the eternal."

One such place in my own life, a favorite place I walk through almost every day, is a small, quiet riverside park not far from my home. Often I settle down there on a park bench and, for a time, rest and view and ponder and pray. Always there is peace, but at times there is even more: a strange flutter of joy which, brief though it is, seems to hint at some vast, ineffable bliss. I am graced, warmed, blessed.

I stand then and, a little stiffly at first, walk on. (The Buddha's last words to his disciples: "Walk on.")

Early in our marriage, after I had made some reference to my house, my car or whatever else, she would gently chide me, "No, my love, it isn't *yours*, it's *ours*." I soon got the message; possessive personal pronouns were to be pluralized.

Now, though, a half-century later, I am having to unlearn all that; I am having to return to premarital forms of expression.

I end a letter, for instance, as I have ended hundreds of others, "We send you our love." But then I am reminded: No, *we* don't send you *our* love; *I* send you *my* love.

Life without her, I find, entails a multitude of such minor adjustments.

$\mathcal{N}$ever—never since infancy, I suppose—have I been so blessed with kindness. Cards and letters, invitations and food, visits and gifts, phone calls and even flowers—day in and day out they keep coming in from every quarter. I am grateful beyond telling.

$\mathcal{W}$e widower friends talked over coffee, he about the staggering immensity of the universe and, it seems, the comparative insignificance of man. How, he wondered, can God possibly care for the individual in so vast a universe?

Familiar lines floated through my mind:

> When I look at your heavens, the work of your fingers,
> the moon and the stars that you have established;
> what are human beings that you are mindful of them,
> mortals that you care for them?
> —Psalm 8:3-4 NRSV

I suggested that as we move up the evolutionary scale, as we move from minerals to mollusks to mice to humankind, we find more and more thinking, feeling, loving.

I went on to comment that on the basis of that progression, it probably follows that beyond humanity, beyond everything, there is infinity itself and, within that infinity, an infinity of love—or Love, a love not governed by limitations of any kind, a Love that embraces every particle in the vast immensity of its beloved creation.

Finally, it seems, the question is this: How can we believe in infinity without believing in an infinity of love?

Knowing her capacity for love, I am convinced that it would not be heaven for my beloved—in fact it would be a minor hell—if she could not continue to be in touch with those she loved so deeply and long and doubtless loves still.

Lines that often come to mind, lines that for me are rich with meaning, are these from the Letter to the Hebrews in the New Testament:

> Therefore, since we are surrounded by so great a cloud of witnesses, let us also lay aside every weight, and sin which clings so

closely, and let us run with perseverance the race that is set before us, looking to Jesus the pioneer and perfecter of our faith.
—Hebrews 12:1-2 rsv

My heart's delight, I am convinced, is one of that invisible "cloud of witnesses," one of that angelic host who are forever near, helping us along the upward way, the celestial way, they have taken themselves.

I often meet him when I am out walking. A slim, dignified gentleman, now verging on eighty, he told me once that he goes out walking, more slowly now, four or five times a day. I complimented him on his self-discipline. He smiled. "I'm trying to stave off decrepitude as long as I can."

Seated in my living room, I have fallen prey to pride; I am thinking of myself in highly flattering terms. But then I look up and see on the bookcase the little Hungarian statuette of a standing, upward gazing Jesus, and seeing that spiritual magnificence, I feel so small, so ashamed of my inward posturing and strutting, that all I can do is breathe an abject prayer for pardon.

$\mathcal{B}$e it pride
in body, mind, or spirit,
inherent in that pride
is contempt.

$\mathcal{A}$s Christians, we remember patriarchs and prophets, and apostles and saints; we remember Jesus of Nazareth and twenty centuries of Christian tradition. We are a people who treasure our heritage. We cherish the past.

Given that vast respect for all that has gone before, can we reasonably believe that those who die, yet live on, differ from us—in fact differ from what they themselves have been—in that they now *reject* their own pasts? Can we believe that now, altogether uncharacteristically, they walk on into the future with never a backward glance?

No, we believe rather that those who have moved on into another life remember us, love us, wait for us. And more, they remain an abiding, an assisting presence throughout our lives until, at the close of life's day, we join them in the glory beyond.

I can take a candle and burn it down until there is nothing left of it. No candle, apparently. Science, though—in its insistence on the indestructibility of matter—maintains that even though the candle has disappeared, it has not been destroyed; it lives on, only not as a candle. It lives on as a trace of carbon, the remains of the wick. It lives on as heat, dissipated but not lost. It lives on as light, a mere pinprick of light, probing out and out forever into the midnight infinity of space.

Surely, though, if God will not permit the loss of even the smallest particle of matter, that same God can be trusted to preserve something infinitely more precious: the human soul. Surely God can be trusted to preserve the essential *you*, the essential *me*.

(After much thought, Alfred North Whitehead, the philosopher, came to the conclusion that God can best be described as "a tender care that nothing be lost.")

In my declining years, the world outside me, my particular world, becomes smaller and smaller. Major accomplishments, heady opportunities, extensive travel and other high adventures are now out of the question. Life now is more localized, more limited, and necessarily so.

A pity? No, not really. Provided I compensate by enlarging my interior world. In fact, right here, I believe, is the essential challenge of old age: finding ways to so expand the world within that ultimately it can accommodate heaven itself.

In life's more difficult times
it helps me to remember that
in view of all He suffered—
and transcended—
I am not entitled to
a painless existence.

Granted, the aging process makes some people more cynical and sour, more selfish and mean, but it is also true that on others it has the opposite effect: it makes them more gentle and humble and kind; it makes them, in their own way, truly beautiful people.

No, generally speaking, I don't pity the aged with their failing bodies and, some of them, their failing minds. On the contrary, I find myself looking beneath the outward deterioration, looking into their minds and hearts, into their yesterdays and tomorrows, and seeing in all that richness an astonishing beauty, a portent perhaps of things to come.

> As a white candle
> In a holy place,
> So is the beauty
> Of an agèd face.
> —Joseph Campbell (Seosamh MacCathmhaoil)[2]

$\mathcal{N}$o sooner had she become a resident in the nursing home than she saw a need and responded: she began portering.

Portering? Portering, I learned, is wheeling those in wheelchairs to and from the dining room, the beauty parlor, the chapel, wheeling them wherever they need to go.

My beloved began portering and kept it up. She kept it up, in fact, until her own mind and body were a shambles, kept it up until she was only weeks away from being in a wheelchair herself.

I think of that shining example and breathe a prayer: *Dear God, help me to keep on giving in small ways as long as I live.*

There are moments, rare moments, when my heart is so filled with gratitude and joy that it feels close to bursting; I fear I may explode.

I thank God for these euphoric moments, but I am also grateful for their brevity. Continuing ecstasy, I think, might be too much to bear.

As I grow old,
my pride lessens,
pride in my abilities,
pride in my body,
pride in my mind.
Perhaps, though,
love moves in only
as pride moves out.

It happened on the day of her father's funeral, she said. After the service, she and her family were being driven to the cemetery in a limousine immediately behind the hearse. It was a desolate time. Everyone in the family was quiet, pensive, sad.

Then, said my friend, she happened to look into the hearse ahead. Through its rear window she saw some daffodils waving gently, and suddenly there came over her a feeling of indescribable elation, that and the utter certainty that her father was alive and supremely well.

It was all she could do, she said, to contain her euphoria. But contain it she did, all the way through the committal service at the cemetery, even though her heart was singing for joy.

She went on to say that ever since that sublime moment she has believed totally that death is not the end. Never again, she said, will she fear death. "I know now that beyond the grave there is everything good. There is life and love and joy."

In the early days of my bereavement, I prayed for her—or tried to pray—but each time, it seemed, there was a strange blockage. As never before, my prayers felt empty, leaden, inert. I sensed no listening ear, no response. Apparently I was not getting through. What was wrong?

Then a question dawned: Could it be that God does not mean us to pray for angels, to pray for those who are beyond our prayers? Could it be that we are required only to *accept*? Accept their presence, their ministrations, their love, and be deeply grateful.

If I could bequeath to those I love only one thing, it would be this: I would bequeath to their memory some of the great hymns of praise and, to their inclination, the will to sing those paeans from their hearts, sing them in joy and desolation both, sing them as long as they live.

This I wish for them above all else, for I deeply believe that nothing—to repeat, *nothing*—so exalts the human spirit as the habitual outpouring of ourselves in praise.

I often hear, "You are in my thoughts and prayers," and I am convinced that those kindly prayers have been more sustaining, more supportive than I can possibly know.

I am also convinced that each day I am blessed in dozens of small, invisible ways, blessed by an unseen hand of which I am utterly unaware.

It was not a moment I had been working and hoping for. It was rather a gift, a gift that came as the most overwhelming surprise of my life. It came not at, say, sunset on an idyllic South Pacific island, a place consistent with the gift itself; it came on a drab downtown street, a place of grimy old buildings and littered gutters.

I was hurrying along, I remember, preoccupied with some minor matter, when suddenly I was so "possessed by love," so engulfed in a vast wave of ecstasy pouring into every part of my being that for a mere minute or two, who knows how long, I was aware only of an ocean, an infinity of love, and, vaguely, the people around me, people I longed to include in its glory. In fact, drawing on the last remnants of propriety, it was all I could do to keep from throwing my arms around those dim, shadowy figures, total strangers, in an attempt to gather them into the dazzling transcendence that had charged my whole universe.

It happened long ago, but ever since that one sublime moment I have known, known with a deep and abiding certainty, that love pulses quietly at the heart of all that is, a love of such overwhelming magnitude that ultimately nothing, not utmost evil and not even death, can prevent it from achieving its marvelous ends.

> One climbs, one sees, one descends; one sees no longer, but one has seen.
> —René Daumel, *Mount Analogue*[3]

$\mathcal{L}$ooking into the face of someone I have long known and loved, I sometimes see not only an older person; I see also the past person, the child I know only from pictures in a family album and the young adult I came to know decades ago; I see too the angelic being, the ultimate person he or she is well on the way to becoming.

In some miniscule way it may be what the Eternal sees in us: the fusion of past, present, and future, the timelessness that is eternity itself.

$\mathcal{H}$e lived in humble circumstances long ago. His father was a carpenter and, at about the age of thirty, he himself became an itinerant preacher. His ministry, however, lasted a mere three years, perhaps even less, and ended in utter disgrace: branded a criminal, he was deserted by all but a handful of followers and died a hideous death.

But today? Today he is widely regarded as the most towering figure in the history of the human race. Even though time can be a merciless discreditor, diminishing and even destroying many a magnificent reputation, twenty centuries of time have only enhanced his stature. Today two billion people worldwide revere him as the most Godlike person who ever lived.

One of his central emphases was that death is not the end. Beyond death, he maintained, there is an eternity of love.

I believe him. I believe him totally. In view of his colossal stature, it would be unthinkable to say he was wrong.

It is now five months since her passing, five months to the day. Rarely now do I have the vivid, the intense sense of her presence that often punctuated the early days of my bereavement.

Is that because, whether from near or far, she knows, knows that I am recovering, knows that I am no longer in such grievous need and she is increasingly free to move on? Perhaps so. But the fact remains: she has by no means entirely left me. Again and again, I find, she is with me. She is with me, a beautiful presence, every time I pause before her picture in our bedroom. She is with me at odd unexpected moments, some casual and some achingly poignant, but with each moment a kiss of a kind, brief and warm, then good-bye—but only for the time being.

The future? I suspect that she will be with me in these rich occasional moments, and with me also in the very depths of my being, as long as I live.

$\mathcal{A}$s an infant, I was cuddled, crooned over, nourished, enjoyed; I was *loved*, loved not because of how much I did or gave but simply because of who and what I was, a small, helpless human being.

I am now an elderly man and, interestingly, my life seems to have come full circle. Again I am being lavished with unearned kindness. Never since earliest childhood have I been so blessed with love.

$\mathcal{F}$rom the day I met her, I was enchanted by her smile, and that radiance, that warmth is the one thing above all others that I look forward to seeing on my arrival Home.

Lines come to mind, the last verse of Cardinal Newman's hymn, "Lead, kindly light":

> So long thy power hath blest me, sure it still will lead me on,
> O'er moor and fen, o'er crag and torrent, till the night is gone;
> And with the morn those angel faces smile
> Which I have loved long since and lost awhile.[4]

In his *Monks of the West*, Charles de Montalembert, the nineteenth-century French Roman Catholic apologist, observed that the finest of those monks, the genuine religious, enjoyed a sublime old age. It was an old age, said de Montalembert, characterized above all else by *benignitas*, a state of extraordinary benevolence, a benevolence that was the final stage in their religious development and, as such, their ultimate vocation, their calling. *Benignitas* was to be added to the earlier monastic virtues of *simplicitas* and *hilaritas*, "thus creating the special significance" of the old man of prayer.

Yes, I would give all I own to end my days in the spirit of that trinity: benevolence, simplicity, joy.

I went to bed late, wakened in the early morning and went back to sleep. Then, on toward dawn, there was the dream. It was the most vivid, the most powerful dream of her I'd had since her death. She was young as I now saw her, young and slim and beautiful, but there was more than youth; there was also an ageless, a timeless quality that was beyond me by far. We stood together, face to face, and, without words, simply *saw* each other, I at least seeing heights and depths, a quality of being that left me speechless.

I was in awe.

We never embraced, never even touched. Yet, amazingly, we had never been closer, never so fused in spirit. How long did this at-onement, this unity last? A minute or two maybe. I don't know. I do know, though, that when shortly I wakened, my eyes were filled with tears. I felt lost, bereft.

Then? Beyond those few tears, there was a marvelous reassurance; there was the profound conviction that somehow all my questions and doubts and fears had been dispelled. I felt *free*, and affirmed and blessed. I was on my way, I knew, to a joyous new life.

It was a near euphoric moment. *Thank you, God*, I murmured. *Thank you, thank you! How can I ever thank you enough?*

PART THREE

Dawn

Throughout my life, and especially in these twilight years, I have been blessed beyond telling by the words of Jesus of Nazareth, the eternal Word, and blessed also by the words of men and women far advanced in the life of the spirit, those who in every age have led the way to the kingdom of God.

Their voices I now share with you, doing so in the hope that many of their affirmations will find a place in your memory, will come to mind again and again, and will, in God's time, help give wings to your soul.

In life, in life beyond death,
God is with us.
We are not alone
Thanks be to God.
    —From the New Creed of The United Church of Canada[1]

Life is eternal; and love is immortal; and death is only a horizon; and a horizon is nothing save the limit of our sight.
    —Rossiter Worthington Raymond[2]

I am standing upon the seashore. A ship at my side spreads her white sails to the morning breeze and starts for the blue ocean. She is an object of beauty and strength, and I stand and watch until at last she hangs like a speck of white cloud just where the sea and sky come down to mingle with each other. Then someone at my side says, "There she goes!"

Gone where? Gone from my sight . . . that is all. She is just as large in mast and hull and spar as she was when she left my side and just as able to bear her load of living freight to the place of destination. Her diminished size is in me, not in her. And just at the moment when someone says, "There she goes!" there are other eyes watching her coming and other voices ready to take up the glad shout, "Here she comes!"

—Henry van Dyke (attr.)[3]

The grave itself is but a covered bridge
Leading from light to light, through a brief darkness.
    —Henry Wadsworth Longfellow[4]

$\mathcal{A}$ man's physical hunger does not prove that that man will get any bread; he may die of starvation on a raft in the Atlantic. But surely a man's hunger does prove that he comes of a race which repairs its body by eating and inhabits a world where eatable substances exist. In the same way, though I do not believe (I wish I did) that my desire for Paradise proves that I shall enjoy it, I think it a pretty good indication that such a thing exists and that some men will. A man may love a woman and not win her; but it would be very odd if the phenomenon called "falling in love" occurred in a sexless world.

—C.S. Lewis[5]

$\mathcal{I}$t is impossible that anything so natural, so necessary, and so universal as death, should ever have been designed by Providence as an evil to mankind.

—Jonathan Swift[6]

$\mathcal{T}$he joy and consolation of our life is realizing that what we have cannot be lost because it is God's.

—Thomas Merton[7]

I lift up my eyes to the hills.
From whence does my help come?
My help comes from the Lord,
who made heaven and earth.

He will not let your foot be moved,
he who keeps you will not slumber.
Behold, he who keeps Israel
will neither slumber nor sleep.

The Lord is your keeper;
the Lord is your shade
on your right hand.
The sun shall not smite you by day,
nor the moon by night.

The Lord will keep you from all evil;
he will keep your life.
The Lord will keep
your going out and your coming in
from this time on and for evermore.
     —Psalm 121 RSV

I was quite certain (of death), and I remember thinking of things and people that I was going to leave; I remember feeling sorry that I hadn't written a masterpiece, that I must leave two people whom I dearly loved, but most of all that I must abandon so many beautiful things, tiny things, the sound of running water, birch trees in the sun, a hot day by the sea, music, reading a good book by the fire, a walk over the hills and so on. Then, with absolute conviction, I was aware that I would be leaving nothing, that whatever I found lovely and of good report I should still enjoy.

—Hugh Walpole[8]

We believe that death does not have the last word. Life has depths in it which death does not touch; it has heights which death cannot reach; it has powers which death cannot quell.

—Samuel H. Miller[9]

$\mathcal{G}$od is our refuge and strength,
a very present help in trouble.
Therefore we will not fear.

—Psalm 46:1-2 RSV

$\mathcal{P}$eople often say they are afraid of death—about, as they sometimes put it, having to be nothing after all these lovely years of being something. When they tell me that, I try to focus the problem more tightly. "Let me see if I understand you," I say. "You're bothered by the thought that you will be non-existent in, say, the year 2075. But tell me something.

"Has it ever occurred to you to worry about the fact that you were likewise non-existent in 1875? Of course it hasn't: for the simple reason that, by the forces of nature alone, you got bravely over that first attack of nothingness and were born. Well, all the Gospel is telling you is that your death—your second bout of nothingness—is going to be even less of a problem than your first. By the power of Jesus' death and resurrection, you will get bravely over that too, and be reborn. In fact, you already have been; so go find something more dangerous to worry about."

—Robert Farrar Capon[10]

I believe that we are created by love and that sooner or later love will draw us up out of our darkness to stand in its exquisite light and see ourselves at last as we really are. The picture I see is of a seed deep in the earth. Somewhere, far up above the weight of darkness pressing down upon the pitiful little seed, is the drawing and the calling of the sun. It seems an impossible journey towards something that has never been seen and cannot be known, but half unconsciously the blind seed puts out roots to steady itself, pushes an imploring hand upwards and starts the struggle. The poor mad poet Christopher Smart said, "the flower glorifies God and parries the adversary." The struggling plant knows as little about the flower he will presently be as he knows about the God he will glorify, but the flower calls to him too as he pushes up through the thick darkness with the adversary clinging to his feet.

—Elizabeth Goudge[11]

Amazing grace, how sweet the sound
That saved a wretch like me!
I once was lost, but now am found,
Was blind, but now I see.

'Twas grace that taught my heart to fear,
and grace my fears relieved;
how precious did that grace appear
the hour I first believed.

Through many dangers, toils, and snares,
I have already come;
'tis grace that brought me safe thus far,
and grace will lead me home.

The Lord has promised good to me,
This word my hope secures;
God will my shield and portion be
As long as life endures.

When we've been there ten thousand years,
bright shining as the sun,
we've no less days to sing God's praise
than when we'd first begun.
   —John Henry Newton[12]

I consider that the sufferings of this present time are not worth comparing with the glory that is to be revealed to us. . . .

We know that in everything God works for good with those who love him, who are called according to his purpose. . . .

Who shall separate us from the love of Christ? Shall tribulation, or distress, or persecution, or famine, or nakedness, or peril, or sword? . . . No, in all these things we are more than conquerors through him who loved us. For I am sure that neither death, nor life, nor angels, nor principalities, nor things present, nor things to come, nor powers, nor height, nor depth, nor anything else in all creation, will be able to separate us from the love of God in Christ Jesus our Lord.

—Romans 8:18, 28, 35, 37-39 RSV

Death is the supreme festival on the road to freedom.
  —Dietrich Bonhoeffer[13]

The leaves fall, fall as if from far away,
like withered things from gardens deep in sky;
they fall with gestures of renunciation.

And through the night the heavy earth falls too,
down from the stars, into the loneliness.

And we all fall. This hand must fall.
Look everywhere: it is the lot of us all.

Yet there is one who holds us as we fall
eternally in his hands' tenderness.
—Rainer Maria Rilke[14]

The eternal God is thy refuge,
and underneath are the everlasting arms.
—Deuteronomy 33:27 KJV

In his love he clothes us, enfolds and embraces us; that tender love completely surrounds us, never to leave us. As I saw it, he is everything that is good.
 —Juliana of Norwich[15]

O Lord, you have made us very small, and we
Bring our years to an end, like a tale that is told.
Help us to remember that beyond our brief day
Is the eternity of your love.
 —Reinhold Niebuhr[16]

The Lord is my shepherd, I shall not want.
He makes me lie down in green pastures;
he leads me beside still waters;
he restores my soul.
He leads me in right paths for his name's sake.
Even though I walk through the darkest valley,
I fear no evil; for you are with me;
your rod and your staff—they comfort me.
You prepare a table before me
in the presence of my enemies;
you anoint my head with oil;
my cup overflows.
Surely goodness and mercy
shall follow me
all the days of my life,
and I shall dwell in the house of the Lord
my whole life long.
  —Psalm 23 NRSV

And he showed me more, a little thing, the size of a hazelnut, on the palm of my hand, round like a ball. I looked at it thoughtfully and wondered, "What is this?" And the answer came, "It is all that is made." I marveled that it continued to exist and did not suddenly disintegrate; it was so small. And again my mind supplied the answer, "It exists, both now and for ever, because God loves it." In short, everything owes its existence to the love of God.

In this "little thing" I saw three truths. The first is that God made it; the second is that God loves it; and the third is that God sustains it. . . . he who is in truth Maker, Keeper, and Lover.

—Juliana of Norwich[17]

O Lord, support us all the day long, until the shadows lengthen and the evening comes, and the busy world is hushed, and the fever of life is over, and our work is done. Then in your mercy grant us a safe lodging, and a holy rest, and peace at the last. Amen.

—John Henry Newman[18]

$\mathcal{L}$et not your hearts be troubled; believe in God, believe also in me. In my Father's house are many rooms; if it were not so, would I have told you that I go to prepare a place for you? And when I go and prepare a place for you, I will come again and will take you to myself, that where I am, you may be also. And you know the way where I am going." Thomas said to him, "Lord, we do not know where you are going; how can we know the way?" Jesus said to him, "I am the way, and the truth, and the life; no one comes to the Father but by me. . . ."

"I will not leave you desolate; I will come to you. Yet a little while, and the world will see me no more, but you will see me; because I live, you will live also. . . ."

"Peace I leave with you; my peace I give to you; not as the world gives do I give to you. Let not your hearts be troubled, neither let them be afraid."

—John 14:1-6, 18-19, 27 RSV

All we know
Of what they do above,
Is that they are happy, and that they love.
    —Edmund Waller[19]

Only when you drink from the river of silence shall you indeed sing.
And when you have reached the mountain top, then you shall begin to climb.
And when the earth shall claim your limbs, then shall you truly dance.
    —Kahlil Gibran[20]

I sigh for the heavenly country,
Where the heavenly people pass,
And the sea is as quiet as a mirror
Of beautiful beautiful glass.

I walk in the heavenly field,
With lilies and poppies bright,
I am dressed in a heavenly coat
Of polished white.

When I walk in the heavenly parkland
My feet on the pasture are bare,
Tall waves the grass, but no harmful
Creature is there.

At night I fly over the housetops,
And stand on the bright moony beams;
Gold are all heaven's rivers
And silver her streams.
    —Stevie Smith[21]

This life is but the passage of a day,
This life is but a pang and all is over;
But in the life to come which fades not away
Every love shall abide and every lover.
    —Christina Rosetti[22]

In the sky
The song of the skylark greets the dawn.
In the fields wet with dew
The scent of violets fills the air.
On such a lovely morning as this
Surely on such a lovely morning as this

Lord Jesus
Came forth
From the tomb.
    —Misuno Genzo[23]

Then I saw a new heaven and a new earth; for the first heaven and the first earth had passed away, and the sea was no more. And I saw the holy city, new Jerusalem, coming down out of heaven from God, prepared as a bride adorned for her husband; and I heard a loud voice from the throne saying,

"Behold, the dwelling of God is with men.

He will dwell with them,

and they shall be his people,

and God himself will be with them;

he will wipe away every tear from their eyes,

and death shall be no more,

neither shall there be mourning nor crying,

nor pain any more,

for the former things have passed away."

—Revelation 21:1-4 RSV

$\mathcal{G}$o forth upon thy journey from this world, O Christian soul,
in the peace of him in whom thou hast believed,
in the name of God the Father, who created thee,
in the name of Jesus, who suffered for thee,
in the name of the Holy Spirit, who strengthened thee.

May the angels and archangels, and all the armies of the heavenly host come to meet thee,
may all the saints of God welcome thee,
may thy portion this day be in gladness and peace,
thy dwelling in Paradise.
Go forth upon thy journey, O Christian soul.
   —Prayer for the dying, from the Roman Ritual[24]

NOTES

Part One: Elegy
1. Dag Hammarskjöld, Leif Sjöberg and W.H. Auden, trans., *Markings* (London: Faber and Faber, 1964), 87.
2. Thomas Merton, *The Sign of Jonas*, in Thomas P. McDonnell, ed., *A Thomas Merton Reader* (New York: Doubleday, Image Books, 1989), 216.
3. Juliana of Norwich, *Revelations of Divine Love*, Ch. 27, Revelation 13, in Angela Partington, ed., *The Oxford Dictionary of Quotations* (Oxford: Oxford University Press, 1992), 382.
4. St. Augustine, in Christopher Herbert, comp., *Words of Comfort* (London: National Society/Church House, 1994), 88.

Part Two: Healing
1. Elie Wiesel, *A Jew Today* (New York: Random House, 1978), 135-36.
2. Joseph Campbell (Seosamh MacCathmhaoil), "Old Woman," *Irishry*, in Tony Augarde, ed., *The Oxford Dictionary of Modern Quotations* (Oxford: Oxford University Press, 1991), 45.
3. René Daumel, *Mount Analogue*, in Marilyn Ferguson, *The Aquarian Conspiracy* (Los Angeles: J.P. Tarcher, 1980), 82-83.
4. John Henry Newman, *Voices United: The Hymn and Worship Book of the United Church of Canada* (Etobicoke, Ont., Canada: The United Church Publishing House, 1996), 640.

Part Three: Dawn
1. *Voices United*, ibid., 918.
2. Rossiter Worthington Raymond, in Maggie Callanan and Patricia Kelley, *Final Gifts: Understanding the Special Awareness, Needs and Communications of the Dying* (New York: Poseidon Press, 1992), 218.
3. Henry van Dyke (attr.), in Phyllis Theroux, ed., *The Book of Eulogies* (New York: Scribner, 1997), 330.
4. Henry Wadsworth Longfellow, *The Golden Legend*, in Margaret Pepper, comp., *The Harper Religious & Inspirational Companion* (London: Harper & Row, 1989), 219.

5. C. S. Lewis, *Transposition and Other Addresses*, Ch. 2 (London: Geoffrey Bles, 1949), 25.

6. Jonathan Swift, "Thoughts on Religion," in D. Enright, ed., *The Oxford Book of Death* (Oxford: Oxford University Press), 29.

7. Thomas Merton, *The Springs of Contemplation*, in Lucinda Vardey, ed., *God in All Worlds* (Toronto: Alfred A. Knopf Canada, 1995), 473.

8. Hugh Walpole, *My Religious Experience*, in Gerald Kennedy, comp., *A Second Reader's Notebook* (New York: Harper & Row, 1959), 98.

9. Samuel H. Miller, in Frederic and Mary Ann Brussat, eds., *Spiritual Literacy* (New York: Scribner, 1996), 368.

10. Robert Farrar Capon, *The Parables of Grace* (Grand Rapids: William B. Eerdman's Publishing Co., 1988), 106, now published as part of *Kingdom, Grace, Judgment*.

11. Elizabeth Goudge, *The Joy of the Snow: An Autobiography* (London: Hodder and Stoughton, 1974), 260-61.

12. John Henry Newton, *Voices United*, ibid., 266.

13. Dietrich Bonhoeffer, *Letters and Papers from Prison*, Eberhard Bethge, ed., (New York: The Macmillan Co., 1971), 376.

14. Rainer Maria Rilke, "Autumn," *Fifty Selected Poems*, C.F. MacIntyre, trans. (Berkeley and San Francisco: University of California Press, 1941), 43.

15. Juliana of Norwich, *Revelations of Divine Love*, in Margaret Pepper, comp., ibid., 206.

16. Reinhold Niebuhr, in *The Gift of Prayer* (New York: Continuum, A Fellowship of Prayer Book, 1995), 232.

17. Juliana of Norwich, in Walter Holden Capps and Wendy M. Wright, eds., *Silent Fire* (New York: Harper & Row, 1978), 99.

18. John Henry Newman, in *The Gift of Prayer*, ibid., 234.

19. Edmund Waller, "Upon the Death of My Lady Rich," in Margaret Pepper, comp., ibid., 309.

20. From *The Prophet* by Kahlil Gilbran, copyright 1923 by Kahlil Gibran and renewed 1951 by Administrators C.T.A. of Kahlil Gibran Estate and Mary G. Gibran. Used by permission of Alfred A. Knopf, a division of Random House, Inc., 81.

21. Stevie Smith, "The Heavenly City," *The Collected Poems of Stevie Smith* (New York: Oxford University Press, 1976), 43.

22. Christina Rosetti, "Saints and Angels," in Margaret Pepper, comp., ibid., 25.

23. Misuno Genzo, in Christopher Herbert, comp., *Words of Comfort*, ibid., 70.

24. From the Roman Ritual, in Christopher Herbert, comp., ibid., 49.